CARDIAC DIET

FOOD LIST

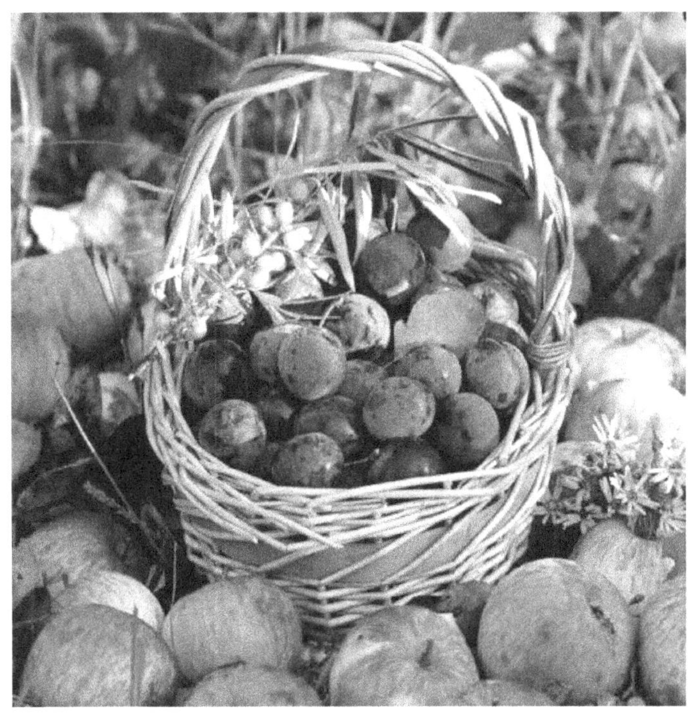

LYSANDRA QUINN

DISCLAIMER

The content within this book reflects my thoughts, experiences, and beliefs. It is meant for informational and entertainment purposes. While I have taken great care to provide accurate information, I cannot guarantee the absolute correctness or applicability of the content to every individual or situation. Please consult with relevant professionals for advice specific to your needs.

OTHER BOOKS MY THE AUTHOR

SLOW COOKER CARDIAC DIET COOKBOOK

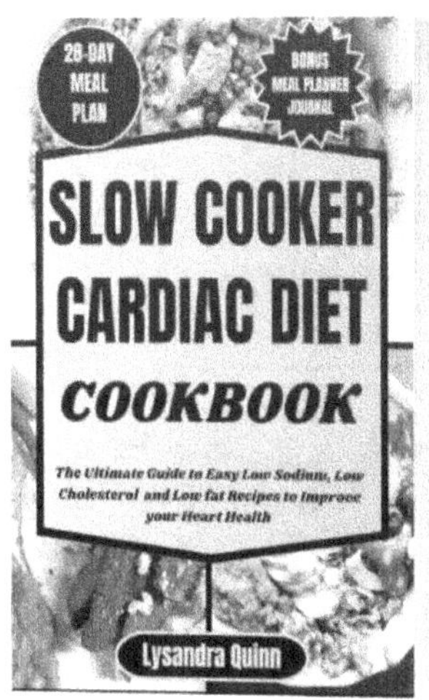

CARDIAC DIET NINJA AIRFYER COOKBOOK

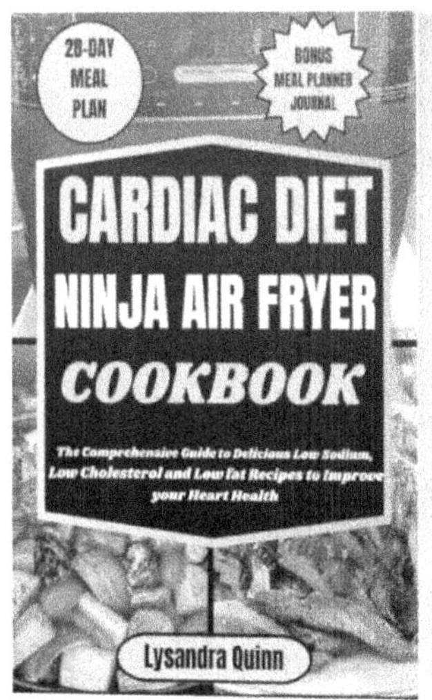

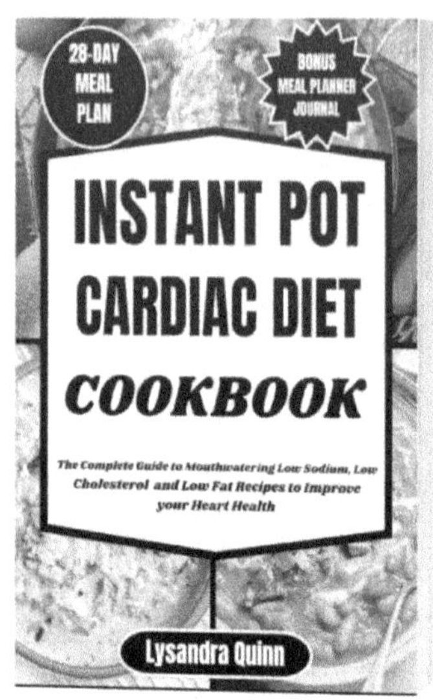
28-DAY MEAL PLAN
BONUS MEAL PLANNER JOURNAL
INSTANT POT
CARDIAC DIET
COOKBOOK
The Complete Guide to Mouthwatering Low Sodium, Low Cholesterol and Low Fat Recipes to Improve your Heart Health
Lysandra Quinn

TABLE OF CONTENTS

INTRODUCTION

In the symphony of life, our hearts play the most delicate and vital notes. Imagine a melody disrupted, a rhythm faltering—a heart in distress. This is a narrative I encountered far too often in my journey as a dietician. Faces etched with worry, eyes reflecting the shadows of health battles, and hearts yearning for a harmonious tune once more.

In my pursuit of understanding the intricate dance of nutrition and heart health, I traversed a landscape of conventional diets and medicinal remedies. I witnessed the frustration etched on the faces of those who had navigated countless food lists, only to find their hearts still whispering a plea for help. It was in this labyrinth of uncertainty that I stumbled upon a revelation—a revelation that sparked the genesis of a journey towards healing, towards a cardiac diet that resonates not just with science but with the very pulse of humanity.

The danger that lurks within the chambers of our hearts is a specter that casts a long shadow upon the paths we tread. Heart disease, a silent predator, stealthily encroaches upon our lives, threatening to disrupt the melody of our existence. It is a foe that pays no heed to age, status, or background, knocking on the doors of the healthy and the seemingly invincible alike.

In the realm of heart health, the stakes are high, and the battleground is the very core of our being. It was amidst this battlefield that I honed my skills as a dietician, a warrior armed not with swords but with the knowledge of nutrition. For twenty-five years, I delved into the science behind cardiac diets, seeking not just a remedy but a revolution in the way we approach heart health.

As the pages of time turned, I bore witness to the transformative power of a carefully curated cardiac diet. This wasn't just a list of foods; it was an elixir that breathed life back into weary hearts. Faces that once mirrored despair now glowed with the radiance of hope and renewed vitality. The stories etched on the canvas of my experience are a testament to the incredible journey from heartache to heart health.

Picture this—a father who, having danced with the shadows of heart disease, now chases after his grandchildren with an exuberance that defies his age. Imagine a woman, once tethered to the chains of medication, now revelling in the liberation of a heart unburdened by the shackles of disease. These are not mere anecdotes; they are the profound echoes of a symphony restored.

The cardiac diet food list I present to you is not a mere collection of ingredients; it is a tapestry woven with the threads of countless stories. It is a guide born not just from clinical expertise but from a deep well of compassion and understanding. This is a food list that transcends the boundaries of conventional wisdom, embracing the nuances of individuality in each heartbeat.

What sets this cardiac diet apart? It is a question that dances on the tip of curiosity, and rightfully so. The answer lies not in the monotony of restriction but in the celebration of variety. This food list is a feast for the heart, a gastronomic journey that marries taste and health in a union that transcends the mundane.

But let us delve beyond the surface. What are the advantages, the benefits that await those who embark on this culinary expedition? Imagine not just a reduction in cholesterol levels but a symphony of nutrients that fortify the very fabric of your cardiovascular system. Envision not just weight management but a culinary experience that embraces the art of nourishment.

This cardiac diet is a compass that guides you towards not just survival, but a life lived in full vibrancy. It is a testament to the fact that the journey to heart health need not be a desolate road, but a scenic route adorned with the colours of flavour and the fragrance of well-being.

As a dietician with a quarter-century of experience, I stand before you not just as a guide but as a witness to the transformative power of conscious eating. This isn't a prescription; it's an invitation to join the ranks of those who have reclaimed their heart's melody.

So, dear reader, as you embark on this literary journey, let the stories within these pages resonate with the rhythm of your own heartbeat. Let the questions that linger in the spaces between the words stir the emotions that dwell within you. Are you ready to not just feed your body but to nourish your heart and soul?

In the realm of heart health, this isn't just a book; it's a love letter to life—a melody composed to the beat of a healthy heart. Welcome to the symphony of well-being.

Contact the Author

Thank you for reading my book! I would love to hear from you, whether you have feedback, questions, or just want to share your thoughts. Your feedback means a lot to me and helps me improve as a writer.

Please don't hesitate to reach out to me through

contactmelysandraquinn@gmail.com

I look forward to connecting with my readers and appreciate your support in this literary journey. Your thoughts and comments are valuable to me.

CHAPTER 1

UNDERSTANDING CARDIAC DIET

A cardiac diet, also known as a heart-healthy diet, is a dietary plan designed to promote heart health and reduce the risk of cardiovascular diseases. This specialized diet focuses on incorporating foods that support optimal heart function while limiting or avoiding those that may contribute to heart-related issues. The goal is to maintain a balance that helps manage factors such as cholesterol levels, blood pressure, and overall cardiovascular well-being.

Key Components of a Cardiac Diet:

Heart-Friendly Fats:

Emphasis on unsaturated fats, found in sources like olive oil, avocados, and nuts.

Limiting saturated fats and trans fats found in fried foods, processed snacks, and fatty meats.

Omega-3 Fatty Acids:

Inclusion of sources rich in omega-3 fatty acids, such as fatty fish (salmon, mackerel, and sardines), flaxseeds, and walnuts.

Omega-3s are known to have anti-inflammatory properties and can contribute to heart health.

Fruits and Vegetables:

High intake of fruits and vegetables, providing essential vitamins, minerals, and antioxidants.

These foods contribute to a well-balanced diet, supporting overall health and cardiovascular function.

Whole Grains:

Incorporation of whole grains like brown rice, quinoa, and whole wheat, which offer fiber and nutrients beneficial for heart health.

Fiber helps in maintaining healthy cholesterol levels and promoting digestive health.

Lean Proteins:

Choosing lean protein sources, such as poultry, fish, legumes, and tofu.

Reducing intake of processed and red meats, which may contain higher levels of unhealthy fats.

Low Sodium Intake:

Monitoring and limiting sodium intake to help manage blood pressure.

Avoiding excessive salt in processed foods and opting for fresh, whole foods.

Moderate Alcohol Consumption:

If alcohol is consumed, do so in moderation.

Moderate alcohol intake has been associated with certain cardiovascular benefits, but excessive consumption can have adverse effects.

Importance of a Heart-Healthy Diet:

Cholesterol Management:

A cardiac diet can help regulate cholesterol levels by reducing the intake of saturated and trans fats, promoting heart health.

Blood Pressure Regulation:

The emphasis on low sodium intake and nutrient-rich foods contributes to the regulation of blood pressure, lowering the risk of hypertension.

Weight Management:

Following a heart-healthy diet supports weight management, reducing the risk of obesity-related cardiovascular issues.

Reduced Inflammation:

Foods rich in antioxidants and omega-3 fatty acids can help combat inflammation, a factor linked to heart disease.

Overall Cardiovascular Health:

The combination of nutrient-dense foods, balanced fats, and mindful eating habits supports the overall well-being of the cardiovascular system.

CHAPTER 2
FRUITS AND VEGETABLES

BERRIES (E.G., BLUEBERRIES, STRAWBERRIES, RASPBERRIES):

Nutritional Information (per cup):

- ✓ Calories: 50-80
- ✓ Fiber: 3-9g
- ✓ Vitamin C: 15-24mg
- ✓ Antioxidants: High

ORANGES:

Nutritional Information (per medium orange):

- ✓ Calories: 62
- ✓ Fiber: 3g
- ✓ Vitamin C: 70mg
- ✓ Potassium: 232mg

APPLES:

Nutritional Information (per medium apple):

- ✓ Calories: 95
- ✓ Fiber: 4g
- ✓ Vitamin C: 14%
- ✓ Antioxidants: Moderate

KIWI:

Nutritional Information (per medium kiwi):

- ✓ Calories: 50
- ✓ Fiber: 2.5g
- ✓ Vitamin C: 71mg
- ✓ Potassium: 215mg

AVOCADO:

Nutritional Information (per half avocado):

- ✓ Calories: 120
- ✓ Fiber: 5g
- ✓ Healthy Fats: 10g
- ✓ Potassium: 345mg

SPINACH:

Nutritional Information (per cup, raw):

- ✓ Calories: 7
- ✓ Fiber: 0.7g
- ✓ Vitamin A: 2813 IU
- ✓ Iron: 0.8mg

KALE:

Nutritional Information (per cup, chopped):

- ✓ Calories: 33
- ✓ Fiber: 2.5g
- ✓ Vitamin K: 547mcg
- ✓ Antioxidants: High

BROCCOLI:

Nutritional Information (per cup, chopped):

- ✓ Calories: 55
- ✓ Fiber: 5g
- ✓ Vitamin C: 81mg
- ✓ Folate: 52mcg

CARROTS:

Nutritional Information (per medium carrot):

- ✓ Calories: 25
- ✓ Fiber: 2g
- ✓ Vitamin A: 10191 IU
- ✓ Potassium: 195mg

SWEET POTATOES:

Nutritional Information (per medium sweet potato):

- ✓ Calories: 103
- ✓ Fiber: 4g
- ✓ Vitamin A: 43896 IU
- ✓ Potassium: 438mg

TOMATOES:

Nutritional Information (per medium tomato):

- ✓ Calories: 22
- ✓ Fiber: 2.2g
- ✓ Vitamin C: 15mg
- ✓ Lycopene: High

BELL PEPPERS (RED, YELLOW, GREEN):

Nutritional Information (per medium pepper):

- ✓ Calories: 25
- ✓ Fiber: 2.5g
- ✓ Vitamin C: 152mg
- ✓ Vitamin A: 3726 IU

GRAPES:

Nutritional Information (per cup):

- ✓ Calories: 104
- ✓ Fiber: 1.4g
- ✓ Antioxidants: Moderate

POMEGRANATE:

Nutritional Information (per cup):

- ✓ Calories: 144
- ✓ Fiber: 6g
- ✓ Vitamin C: 10.2mg
- ✓ Antioxidants: High

CAULIFLOWER:

Nutritional Information (per cup, chopped):

- ✓ Calories: 27
- ✓ Fiber: 2.1g
- ✓ Vitamin C: 51mg
- ✓ Folate: 55mcg

CELERY:

Nutritional Information (per cup):

- ✓ Calories: 16
- ✓ Fiber: 1.6g
- ✓ Vitamin K: 30mcg
- ✓ Potassium: 263mg

CUCUMBER:

Nutritional Information (per cup, sliced):

- ✓ Calories: 16
- ✓ Fiber: 0.5g
- ✓ Vitamin K: 19mcg
- ✓ Hydration: High

GARLIC:

Nutritional Information (per clove):

- ✓ Calories: 4
- ✓ Vitamin C: 1%
- ✓ Antioxidants: Allicin

ONIONS:

Nutritional Information (per medium onion):

- ✓ Calories: 46
- ✓ Fiber: 3g
- ✓ Vitamin C: 11mg
- ✓ Quercetin: Moderate

BEETS:

Nutritional Information (per cup, cooked):

- ✓ Calories: 59
- ✓ Fiber: 3.8g
- ✓ Folate: 136mcg
- ✓ Potassium: 442mg

CHAPTER 3

WHOLE GRAINS

QUINOA:

Nutritional Information (per cup, cooked):

- ✓ Calories: 222
- ✓ Protein: 8g
- ✓ Fiber: 5g
- ✓ Magnesium: 118mg

OATS:

Nutritional Information (per cup, cooked):

- ✓ Calories: 147
- ✓ Protein: 6g
- ✓ Fiber: 4g
- ✓ Beta-glucans: Supportive of heart health

BROWN RICE:

Nutritional Information (per cup, cooked):

- ✓ Calories: 215
- ✓ Protein: 5g
- ✓ Fiber: 3.5g
- ✓ Magnesium: 83mg

BARLEY:

Nutritional Information (per cup, cooked):

- ✓ Calories: 193
- ✓ Protein: 3.5g
- ✓ Fiber: 6g
- ✓ Beta-glucans: Supportive of heart health

BUCKWHEAT:

Nutritional Information (per cup, cooked):

- ✓ Calories: 155
- ✓ Protein: 6g
- ✓ Fiber: 5g
- ✓ Magnesium: 86mg

WHOLE WHEAT:

Nutritional Information (per cup, cooked):

- ✓ Calories: 173
- ✓ Protein: 6.5g
- ✓ Fiber: 4.5g
- ✓ Magnesium: 55mg

FARRO:

Nutritional Information (per cup, cooked):

- ✓ Calories: 220
- ✓ Protein: 8g
- ✓ Fiber: 8g
- ✓ Magnesium: 68mg

MILLET:

Nutritional Information (per cup, cooked):

- ✓ Calories: 207
- ✓ Protein: 6g
- ✓ Fiber: 2.3g
- ✓ Magnesium: 76mg

AMARANTH:

Nutritional Information (per cup, cooked):

- ✓ Calories: 251
- ✓ Protein: 9g
- ✓ Fiber: 5g
- ✓ Calcium: 116mg

WILD RICE:

Nutritional Information (per cup, cooked):

- ✓ Calories: 166
- ✓ Protein: 6.5g
- ✓ Fiber: 3g
- ✓ Magnesium: 52mg

CHPATER 4

LEAN PROTEINS

CHICKEN BREAST:

Nutritional Information (per 3.5 oz, cooked):

- ✓ Calories: 165
- ✓ Protein: 31g
- ✓ Total Fat: 3.6g
- ✓ Saturated Fat: 1g

TURKEY (GROUND OR BREAST):

Nutritional Information (per 3.5 oz, cooked):

- ✓ Calories: 135
- ✓ Protein: 30g
- ✓ Total Fat: 1g
- ✓ Saturated Fat: 0.3g

FISH (SALMON, MACKEREL, TROUT):

Nutritional Information (per 3.5 oz, cooked):

- ✓ Calories: 206
- ✓ Protein: 22g
- ✓ Total Fat: 13g
- ✓ Omega-3 Fatty Acids: High

TOFU:

Nutritional Information (per 3.5 oz, cooked):

- ✓ Calories: 144
- ✓ Protein: 15g
- ✓ Total Fat: 8g
- ✓ Iron: 2.1mg

BEANS (BLACK BEANS, KIDNEY BEANS, CHICKPEAS):

Nutritional Information (per cup, cooked):

- ✓ Calories: 220-260
- ✓ Protein: 15g
- ✓ Total Fat: 1-2g
- ✓ Fiber: 15g

LEAN BEEF (SIRLOIN OR TENDERLOIN):

Nutritional Information (per 3.5 oz, cooked):

- ✓ Calories: 250
- ✓ Protein: 26g
- ✓ Total Fat: 17g
- ✓ Saturated Fat: 6.5g

PORK TENDERLOIN:

Nutritional Information (per 3.5 oz, cooked):

- ✓ Calories: 143
- ✓ Protein: 26g
- ✓ Total Fat: 4g
- ✓ Saturated Fat: 1g

EGGS:

Nutritional Information (per large egg):

- ✓ Calories: 70
- ✓ Protein: 6g
- ✓ Total Fat: 5g
- ✓ Choline: 147mg

GREEK YOGURT (LOW-FAT OR FAT-FREE):

Nutritional Information (per cup):

- ✓ Calories: 100
- ✓ Protein: 17g
- ✓ Total Fat: 0g
- ✓ Calcium: 200mg

SKINLESS TURKEY OR CHICKEN SAUSAGES:

Nutritional Information (per 3.5 oz, cooked):

- ✓ Calories: 140-170
- ✓ Protein: 15-20g
- ✓ Total Fat: 8-10g
- ✓ Sodium: 400-600mg

CHPATER 5

DAIRY AND ALTERNATIVES

LOW-FAT OR FAT-FREE MILK:

Nutritional Information (per cup):

- ✓ Calories: 80-90
- ✓ Protein: 8g
- ✓ Total Fat: 0-1g
- ✓ Calcium: 300mg

CHEESE (PART-SKIM MOZZARELLA OR FETA):

Nutritional Information (per ounce):

- ✓ Calories: 70-80
- ✓ Protein: 6-7g
- ✓ Total Fat: 4-6g
- ✓ Calcium: 200mg

COTTAGE CHEESE (LOW-FAT OR FAT-FREE):

Nutritional Information (per cup):

- ✓ Calories: 210
- ✓ Protein: 28g
- ✓ Total Fat: 1g
- ✓ Calcium: 220mg

ALMOND MILK (UNSWEETENED):

Nutritional Information (per cup):

- ✓ Calories: 30
- ✓ Protein: 1g
- ✓ Total Fat: 2.5g
- ✓ Calcium: 450mg (fortified)

SOY MILK (UNSWEETENED):

Nutritional Information (per cup):

- ✓ Calories: 80
- ✓ Protein: 7g
- ✓ Total Fat: 4g
- ✓ Calcium: 300mg (fortified)

OAT MILK (UNSWEETENED):

Nutritional Information (per cup):

- ✓ Calories: 80-120
- ✓ Protein: 2-4g
- ✓ Total Fat: 1-5g
- ✓ Calcium: Varies (fortified)

FLAX MILK (UNSWEETENED):

Nutritional Information (per cup):

- ✓ Calories: 25-60
- ✓ Protein: 0-1g
- ✓ Total Fat: 2.5-6g
- ✓ Calcium: Varies (fortified)

PROBIOTIC YOGURT DRINKS (LOW-FAT OR DAIRY-FREE):

Nutritional Information (per cup):

- ✓ Calories: 50-80
- ✓ Protein: 1-3g
- ✓ Total Fat: 0-3g
- ✓ Calcium: Varies

RICOTTA CHEESE (PART-SKIM):

Nutritional Information (per ounce):

- ✓ Calories: 50
- ✓ Protein: 3g
- ✓ Total Fat: 4g
- ✓ Calcium: 150mg

SKIM MILK (NON-FAT):

Nutritional Information (per cup):

- ✓ Calories: 80
- ✓ Protein: 8g
- ✓ Total Fat: 0g
- ✓ Calcium: 300mg

CHAPTER 6

NUTS AND SEEDS

ALMONDS:

Nutritional Information (per ounce, about 23 almonds):

- ✓ Calories: 160
- ✓ Protein: 6g
- ✓ Total Fat: 14g
- ✓ Fiber: 3.5g

WALNUTS:

Nutritional Information (per ounce, about 14 halves):

- ✓ Calories: 185
- ✓ Protein: 4.3g
- ✓ Total Fat: 18.5g
- ✓ Omega-3 Fatty Acids: High

FLAXSEEDS:

Nutritional Information (per tablespoon, ground):

- ✓ Calories: 37
- ✓ Protein: 1.3g
- ✓ Total Fat: 3g
- ✓ Omega-3 Fatty Acids: High

CHIA SEEDS:

Nutritional Information (per ounce, about 2 tablespoons):

- ✓ Calories: 138
- ✓ Protein: 4.7g
- ✓ Total Fat: 8.7g
- ✓ Omega-3 Fatty Acids: High

PUMPKIN SEEDS (PEPITAS):

- ✓ **Nutritional Information (per ounce):**
- ✓ Calories: 151
- ✓ Protein: 7g
- ✓ Total Fat: 13g
- ✓ Magnesium: 150mg

SUNFLOWER SEEDS:

Nutritional Information (per ounce):

- ✓ Calories: 164
- ✓ Protein: 5.5g
- ✓ Total Fat: 14g
- ✓ Vitamin E: 7.4mg

CASHEWS:

Nutritional Information (per ounce, about 18 cashews):

- ✓ Calories: 157
- ✓ Protein: 5g
- ✓ Total Fat: 12g
- ✓ Magnesium: 83mg

BRAZIL NUTS:

Nutritional Information (per ounce, about 6 nuts):

- ✓ Calories: 182
- ✓ Protein: 4g
- ✓ Total Fat: 19g
- ✓ Selenium: Very high (excellent for thyroid function)

PISTACHIOS:

Nutritional Information (per ounce, about 49 kernels):

- ✓ Calories: 159
- ✓ Protein: 6g
- ✓ Total Fat: 13g
- ✓ Fiber: 3g

HAZELNUTS (FILBERTS):

Nutritional Information (per ounce, about 21 nuts):

- ✓ Calories: 178
- ✓ Protein: 4g
- ✓ Total Fat: 17g
- ✓ Vitamin E: 4.3mg

CHAPTER 7

FOODS TO AVOID OR LIMIT

PROCESSED MEATS (BACON, SAUSAGES, HOT DOGS):

Nutritional Information (per 2 slices of bacon):

- ✓ Calories: 84
- ✓ Total Fat: 7g
- ✓ Saturated Fat: 2.5g
- ✓ Sodium: 346mg

FRIED FOODS (FRENCH FRIES, FRIED CHICKEN):

Nutritional Information (per medium serving of French fries):

- ✓ Calories: 365
- ✓ Total Fat: 17g
- ✓ Saturated Fat: 2.3g
- ✓ Sodium: 163mg

PROCESSED SNACK FOODS (CHIPS, PRETZELS):

Nutritional Information (per 1 oz of potato chips):

- ✓ Calories: 152
- ✓ Total Fat: 10g
- ✓ Saturated Fat: 3g
- ✓ Sodium: 136mg

PACKAGED PASTRIES (DOUGHNUTS, PASTRIES):

Nutritional Information (per glazed doughnut):

- ✓ Calories: 195
- ✓ Total Fat: 12g
- ✓ Saturated Fat: 6g
- ✓ Added Sugars: 12g.

FULL-FAT DAIRY PRODUCTS (WHOLE MILK, FULL-FAT CHEESE):

Nutritional Information (per cup of whole milk):

- ✓ Calories: 149
- ✓ Total Fat: 8g
- ✓ Saturated Fat: 4.6g
- ✓ Cholesterol: 24mg

HIGH-SUGAR CEREALS:

Nutritional Information (per cup of a sugary cereal):

- ✓ Calories: Varies
- ✓ Total Fat: Varies
- ✓ Added Sugars: Varies
- ✓ Fiber: Varies

SUGARY BEVERAGES (SODAS, FRUIT JUICES):

Nutritional Information (per 12 oz soda):

- ✓ Calories: 140
- ✓ Added Sugars: 39g.
- ✓ Sodium: 30mg

PROCESSED AND RED MEATS (BURGERS, PROCESSED DELI MEATS):

Nutritional Information (per 3 oz beef burger):

- ✓ Calories: 220
- ✓ Total Fat: 17g
- ✓ Saturated Fat: 6.5g
- ✓ Sodium: 70mg

WHOLE MILK YOGURT WITH ADDED SUGARS:

Nutritional Information (per 6 oz serving):

- ✓ Calories: 150
- ✓ Total Fat: 6g
- ✓ Added Sugars: 20g.
- ✓ Protein: 8g

HIGH-SODIUM SOUPS AND BROTHS:

Nutritional Information (per cup of canned soup):

- ✓ Calories: Varies
- ✓ Total Fat: Varies
- ✓ Sodium: Varies
- ✓ Protein: Varies

WHITE BREAD AND BAKERY GOODS:

Nutritional Information (per slice of white bread):

- ✓ Calories: 79
- ✓ Total Fat: 1g
- ✓ Sodium: 147mg
- ✓ Carbohydrates: 14g

COMMERCIALLY BAKED GOODS (COOKIES, PASTRIES):

Nutritional Information (per chocolate chip cookie):

- ✓ Calories: 50
- ✓ Total Fat: 2.5g
- ✓ Added Sugars: 5g.
- ✓ Sodium: 25mg

CANNED VEGETABLES WITH ADDED SALT:

Nutritional Information (per cup of canned green beans):

- ✓ Calories: 38
- ✓ Total Fat: 0g
- ✓ Sodium: 364mg
- ✓ Fiber: 4g

HIGH-FAT SALAD DRESSINGS:

Nutritional Information (per 2 tbsp of creamy dressing):

- ✓ Calories: 140
- ✓ Total Fat: 14g
- ✓ Saturated Fat: 2g
- ✓ Sodium: 260mg

ICE CREAM AND FROZEN DESSERTS:

Nutritional Information (per 1/2 cup vanilla ice cream):

- ✓ Calories: 137
- ✓ Total Fat: 7g
- ✓ Saturated Fat: 4g
- ✓ Added Sugars: 14g.

CANNED FRUIT IN SYRUP:

Nutritional Information (per cup of canned peaches in syrup):

- ✓ Calories: 160
- ✓ Total Fat: 0g
- ✓ Added Sugars: 25g.
- ✓ Fiber: 2.5g

MARGARINE AND TRANS FAT-CONTAINING SPREADS:

Nutritional Information (per tablespoon of margarine):

- ✓ Calories: 102
- ✓ Total Fat: 12g
- ✓ Trans Fat: 3g
- ✓ Sodium: 107mg

EXCESSIVE ALCOHOL:

Nutritional Information (per 5 oz glass of red wine):

- ✓ Calories: 125
- ✓ Total Carbohydrates: 4g
- ✓ Alcohol Content: 15g

HIGHLY PROCESSED FAST FOOD:

Nutritional Information (per medium-sized fast-food burger):

- ✓ Calories: 250-400 (varies widely)
- ✓ Total Fat: 10-25g (varies widely)
- ✓ Sodium: 500-1000mg (varies widely)

ENERGY DRINKS:

Nutritional Information (per 8 oz serving):

- ✓ Calories: 110
- ✓ Total Carbohydrates: 28g
- ✓ Added Sugars: 27g.
- ✓ Caffeine: Varies (usually high)

CONCLUSION

As our journey through the tapestry of heart health reaches its final crescendo, let us pause and reflect on the harmonies we have discovered within these pages. We've navigated the corridors of danger, danced with the shadows of uncertainty, and emerged into the radiant light of hope. This cardiac diet food list is not just a guide; it is a compass that directs us towards a life steeped in the vibrant hues of well-being.

In the symphony of life, where our hearts play the most poignant notes, the importance of nurturing our cardiovascular health cannot be overstated. As you close this chapter, envision a future where your heart beats not just in survival but in the exhilarating dance of vitality. Let the flavors of these recipes linger on your palate, a reminder that conscious eating is not a chore but a celebration—a celebration of life, love, and longevity.

I implore you, dear reader, to embrace this cardiac diet not as a prescription but as a pledge to yourself—a pledge to savor each moment, to revel in the nourishment that transcends the plate and touches the very essence of your being. Let the stories shared in these pages serve as beacons of inspiration, guiding you towards a heart that beats with resilience and joy.

Our hearts, like well-composed symphonies, yearn for resonance and harmony. This cardiac diet food list is the conductor of that symphony, orchestrating a melody that echoes with the vitality of a life well-lived. As the final notes linger in the air, I invite you to share your own journey. Your feedback is not just valuable; it is the encore, the continuation of this symphony.

In your reflections, find the courage to pen your thoughts, the highs, the lows, and the moments of revelation. Let your words be a part of the ongoing narrative, a chorus that adds depth to the collective experience. Your feedback is not just a critique; it is a conversation, a dialogue that propels us forward in our shared pursuit of heart health.

As a dietician who has traversed the realms of nutrition for a quarter of a century, I stand here not with a conclusion but with an invitation—an invitation to join hands in the ongoing symphony of well-being. Your thoughts, your experiences, your feedback—they are the notes that harmonize with the melody of this journey.

So, as you embark on the practical application of these recipes, as you savor the flavors and reap the benefits, let your voice be heard. Together, let us compose a chorus of health, resilience, and joy—a symphony that echoes through the corridors of time.

In closing, thank you for entrusting me with a part of your journey. May your heart continue to beat with the rhythm of vitality, and may this cardiac diet be the soundtrack to a life abundantly lived. Until we meet again, let the symphony of well-being play on.

BONUS

10 CARDIAC DIET RECIPES

Baked Lemon Herb Salmon:

Cooking Time: 20 minutes

Serving: 4

Ingredients:

- ✓ 4 salmon fillets
- ✓ 2 tbsp olive oil
- ✓ 1 lemon (sliced)
- ✓ Fresh herbs (rosemary, thyme)

Instructions:

1. Preheat oven to 400°F.
2. Place salmon on a baking sheet.
3. Drizzle with olive oil, add lemon slices, and sprinkle with herbs.
4. Bake for 15 minutes.

Nutritional Info:

250 calories, 0g carbs, 30g protein, 14g fat, 0g fiber

Quinoa and Vegetable Stuffed Peppers:

Cooking Time: 30 minutes

Serving: 6

Ingredients:

- ✓ 1 cup quinoa (cooked)
- ✓ 6 bell peppers (halved)
- ✓ 1 cup black beans (cooked)
- ✓ 1 cup corn kernels

Instructions:

1. Preheat oven to 375°F.
2. Mix quinoa, black beans, and corn. Stuff peppers.
3. Bake for 25 minutes.

Nutritional Info:

180 calories, 35g carbs, 7g protein, 2g fat, 6g fiber

Grilled Chicken and Vegetable Skewers:

Cooking Time: 15 minutes

Serving: 4

Ingredients:

- ✓ 1 lb chicken breast (cubed)
- ✓ Assorted vegetables (bell peppers, zucchini, cherry tomatoes)
- ✓ Olive oil, garlic, lemon juice

Instructions:

1. Marinate chicken in olive oil, garlic, and lemon juice.
2. Thread chicken and vegetables onto skewers.
3. Grill for 10-12 minutes.

Nutritional Info:

220 calories, 5g carbs, 30g protein, 9g fat, 2g fiber

Mango Avocado Quinoa Salad:

Prep Time: 15 minutes

Serving: 4

Ingredients:

- ✓ 1 cup quinoa (cooked)
- ✓ 1 ripe mango (diced)
- ✓ 1 avocado (diced)
- ✓ Cherry tomatoes, red onion, cilantro

Instructions:

1. Combine quinoa, mango, avocado, tomatoes, onion, and cilantro.
2. Toss with olive oil and lemon juice.

Nutritional Info:

220 calories, 30g carbs, 4g protein, 10g fat, 6g fiber

Turkey and Vegetable Stir-Fry:

Cooking Time: 20 minutes

Serving: 4

Ingredients:

- ✓ 1 lb ground turkey
- ✓ Broccoli, bell peppers, snap peas
- ✓ Low-sodium soy sauce, ginger, garlic

Instructions:

1. Brown turkey in a skillet.
2. Add vegetables, soy sauce, ginger, and garlic.
3. Stir-fry until vegetables are tender.

Nutritional Info:

250 calories, 15g carbs, 25g protein, 10g fat, 5g fiber

Lentil and Vegetable Soup:

Cooking Time: 45 minutes

Serving: 6

Ingredients:

- ✓ 1 cup lentils (rinsed)
- ✓ Carrots, celery, onion, garlic
- ✓ Low-sodium vegetable broth, cumin, coriander

Instructions:

1. Sauté vegetables and spices in a pot.
2. Add lentils and broth. Simmer for 30 minutes.

Nutritional Info:

180 calories, 30g carbs, 12g protein, 1g fat, 10g fiber

Spinach and Feta Stuffed Chicken Breast:

Cooking Time: 30 minutes

Serving: 4

Ingredients:

- ✓ 4 chicken breasts
- ✓ Spinach, feta cheese, garlic
- ✓ Olive oil, lemon juice

Instructions:

1. Butterfly chicken breasts.
2. Sauté spinach and garlic. Stuff chicken with spinach and feta.
3. Bake for 25 minutes.

Nutritional Info:

280 calories, 2g carbs, 35g protein, 15g fat, 1g fiber

Brown Rice and Black Bean Bowl:

Cooking Time: 25 minutes

Serving: 4

Ingredients:

- ✓ 2 cups brown rice (cooked)
- ✓ 1 can black beans (rinsed)
- ✓ Avocado, cherry tomatoes, cilantro
- ✓ Lime juice, cumin, salt

Instructions:

1. Mix rice, black beans, avocado, tomatoes, and cilantro.
2. Season with lime juice, cumin, and salt.

Nutritional Info:

240 calories, 45g carbs, 8g protein, 5g fat, 8g fiber

Oven-Baked Cod with Herbs:

Cooking Time: 20 minutes

Serving: 2

Ingredients:

- ✓ 2 cod fillets
- ✓ Fresh herbs (parsley, dill)
- ✓ Lemon juice, olive oil, garlic

Instructions:

1. Preheat oven to 400°F.
2. Place cod in a baking dish. Sprinkle with herbs, lemon juice, and olive oil.
3. Bake for 15 minutes.

Nutritional Info:

180 calories, 0g carbs, 30g protein, 7g fat, 0g fiber

Veggie and Hummus Wrap:

Prep Time: 15 minutes

Serving: 2

Ingredients:

- ✓ Whole wheat wraps
- ✓ Hummus, cucumber, bell peppers, spinach
- ✓ Feta cheese, olives (optional)

Instructions:

1. Spread hummus on wraps.
2. Fill it with sliced veggies and cheese.

Nutritional Info:

280 calories, 40g carbs, 10g protein, 10g fat, 8g fiber